# Fasting For The Carnivore Diet

# Copyright

# Table of Contents

# Introduction

Thank you for purchasing *Fasting for the Carnivore Diet!* We hope that this book will answer all of the questions you have regarding fasting and the carnivore diet. If you've bought this book, maybe you're curious to learn more about fasting and the new trend you've heard about. Despite being a ritual that has existed since the beginning of our civilization, intermittent fasting has become more and more popular in recent years. People are learning the great secret about fasting – that if you give up food for a little while, you can actually improve your health! You may even extend your lifespan!

This book is all about giving you a thorough introduction to fasting and exactly what it entails. That means the history behind it, the benefits and science of fasting, and how to begin a ritual of fasting in your routine. Fasting can be tough and overwhelming – giving up something always is. But when we see the history of fasting and realize its deep roots in society, we see that our bodies can make this adjustment, especially when we see the powerful ways it could benefit our health!

Fasting is often criticized as an "extreme" measure to losing weight. But, in this book, we go over how, anthropologically, in our history as a society, our ancestors had to adjust and fast during times of uncertainty and famine. Even the Father of Modern Medicine, the Greek doctor Hippocrates, urged fasting as a method of easing sickness and promoting wellness. Aristotle, Plato, Benjamin Franklin... so many great minds urged fasting as a way of promoting health and ensuring you didn't overeat. Fasting is often thought of in a spiritual context, so we see how many world religions include fasting in their religious calendar. You've probably heard of the holidays like Lent, Ramadan, or Yom Kippur – all involve fasting!

Some of the most astonishing information people learn is just how many health benefits fasting can possibly bring  By sacrificing a little now, you're gaining the potential of a healthier and longer life – which is better than even losing a few pounds! Whether it's possibly preventing cancer or neurodegenerative diseases, improving mental focus and acuity, reducing cardiovascular risk factors like blood pressure and cholesterol, or simply improving your mood and giving you more energy, fasting could be just what you need. Pre-diabetic people consider it as a great option to stabilize blood sugar levels and prevent the body from becoming insulin resistant. Along with all that, fasting can also help you get rid of that stubborn weight you can't get rid of. By abstaining from food, you're allowing your body to harness energy it already has from fat it has stored away. This means burning fat for fuel and losing weight at the same time!

Before making any changes to your diet or routine, it's important that you first talk to your doctor to assure you are able to fast and do not pose any health concerns. If you have a severe medical condition or are required to take medication or insulin throughout the day, then fasting may not be right for you. People who have a history with eating disorders, women who are pregnant, breastfeeding or trying to conceive, and children under 13 years old should not fast as well. It's important that you first talk to your doctor to ensure that fasting is an acceptable option for you.

Once you have the green light, we are here to help you with the process! We will provide information on the carnivore diet to help you during your eating windows and give you some tips on how to ease into a routine of fasting. Sometimes, going slowly by simply cutting out snacks and skipping a meal or two is just what your body needs to get adjusted. Along with those tips, we will provide many others to help you become comfortable with fasting and make your fasting window more manageable. The more prepared you are, the greater your chances for success!

There are plenty of books on this subject on the market, so thanks again for choosing this one! We hope this book answers your questions regarding fasting and how it could be beneficial for you!

# Chapter 1

# Introducing Fasting & Its History

Most people tend to think of the term "fasting" as a religious ritual that only the highly religious followers partake in. Fasting does have roots in almost all world religions, but it's also become popular again as a method of fasting intermittently to gain many health benefits. Fasting was something ancient civilizations took part in not only for spiritual benefits but also for improving their health and avoiding overeating. Studies have shown that fasting can successfully help you lose weight, improve mental concentration and alertness, reduce inflammation and blood pressure, and prevent insulin resistance that can lead to diabetes. With studies linking fasting to many of these health benefits, it's easy to see why intermittent fasting has become a more recent trend.

In recent generations, due to the abundance of wealth and easiness of getting food, we are treating yourself to multiple meals of days – plus snacks! This presence of food at every hour of the day has made it, so we are not able to endure a period of time without food as our ancestors did. They were much more used to periods of "feast or famine" and often had to skip meals or fast in order to conserve or let other members of the family eat.

One of the problems with constantly eating throughout the day is that your body is only burning carbohydrates for quick fuel instead of burning fat, which takes a longer time to burn. Our bodies already have fat stored in reserve, but it doesn't get a chance to burn it for fuel because we're constantly replenishing the body with food throughout the body. By simply extending the time between meals, you're giving your body the opportunity to burn energy it already has, which can help you lose weight.

In fact, when we are constantly eating and having snacks throughout the day, the body's insulin levels rise as we consume fat or carbohydrates. The chemical process is actually called "De Novo Lipogenesis," which translates to "making fat from new." Basically, when you have a meal, the body needs anywhere from 3 to 6 hours to digest that meal. It stores away that energy until it is triggered to burn the fuel. With fasting, the body starts to signal that there's a shortage of incoming food. The blood sugar levels decrease, and the body realizes it needs to use glucose from storage that it already has saved. You end up using the energy you already had stored away instead of constantly eating more food.

Anthropologically speaking, that's how our bodies are designed and how our ancestors adjusted during periods of famine or drought. For primitive societies that were hunters and gatherers, they would have to adjust and train their body for times when food was scarce. Did their bodies go into starvation mode simply because of a missed meal or two? Of course not. They had to learn to adjust and maybe sacrifice food during difficult times so that children or the elderly could eat instead. Skipping a meal didn't mean they went hungry. It just gave their body time to use the reserves it had stored away for a "rainy day" where food was scarce. When it comes to natural selection, evolutionarily speaking, the individuals who are able to resist hunger and function for longer periods of time without food would be more adept at surviving.

Critics of fasting will try to equate it with starvation and say you are going to extreme levels just to lose weight. But fasting is a ritual that has existed since the beginning of time, whether for evolutionary reasons or for religious observance. Equating it with starvation is wrong and actually disrespectful to those who are struggling to have enough to meat. Starvation means not knowing where your next meal is coming from and having to suffer in hunger and sorrow while patiently waiting. Fasting is voluntarily giving up food for your own reasons - whether that's health-related or religious reasons. Whether it's extending your window of time without food for a few hours or a day, you're confident in the knowledge that you have a meal waiting for you and you get to decide when you will eat it.

Intermittent fasting has become a popular trend in terms of dieting because of the flexibility it provides. It's all about your comfort level and how you choose to make the decision about your fasting versus eating time. The goal of including fasting in your routine is to become healthier overall so even in your allotted eating window, you should be eating healthy and filling foods full of energy, protein, and carbohydrates to make it through your fasting window. During your fasting window, you should not eat any food though beverages such as water, tea, or coffee are allowed as long as they do not contain calories. Caffeine is actually encouraged because it dulls the body's hunger pangs and makes you feel fuller for longer. That's how sometimes after you have a few cups of coffee, you feel less hungry and can often delay your meal or snack time.

How long do you want to go without food? That's up to you! People wrongly assume fasting has to go on for a period of days, or that you're testing your body to its last limit. Not true! Many people will have block windows that they will go without food. Whether it's a 12-hour fast, a 16-hour fast, an 18-hour, or a 1-day fast, it's completely up to you to be in control of your fasting window. Those may seem like

impossible windows of time to go
without food, but most people are often
fasting 12 hours without realizing it!
Let's say you have dinner every night by
7:30 PM and you only have a cup of tea
before bed. The next morning you might
be up by 6:30 AM, but with your busy
morning routine and commute, you only
have a cup of coffee before being able to
grab breakfast around 8 AM. That's a 12-
hour window where you have not eaten.
What intermittent fasting does is give
people the incentive of health benefits
and weight loss to push that window a
little longer. For example, if you manage
to just have morning coffee and delay
your breakfast until 11:30 AM, that's a
16-hour fasting window you've
completed! It's all about adjusting your
day, and you're eating habits so that you
get the benefits you want.

## *The History of Fasting*

Fasting has been something prescribed and written about from people as early as Hippocrates, who is coined the Father of Modern Medicine. He wrote that "To eat when you are sick is to feed your illness." It explains the body's natural tendency to be unable to eat when you are sick and how you feel like you've lost your appetite, or your taste buds have changed. Doctors in Greek society often prescribed fasting for patients who were sick. Great thinkers like Plato and Aristotle were also fans of fasting and feared overeating or consuming food in excess. As medicine evolved in the West, Philip Paracelsus also labeled fasting as the "physician within." He was another doctor who was considered one of the fathers of Western medicine along with Galen and Hippocrates. Even Benjamin Franklin wrote, "The best of all

medicines is resting and fasting." Great
thinkers of the time thought of fasting as
a healing technique to aid speedy
recovery and that it was always best to
limit excess intake of food.

But the most established ritual of
fasting is probably from its roots in
nearly all major world religions. Nearly
each one shares a belief that fasting has
redeeming spiritual benefits and the
power of healing. Whether that purpose
is to ask forgiveness for sins or to purify
your soul, nearly all organized world
religions ask their followers to give up
food (and sometimes even water!) to
follow an ancient ritual of spirituality.

Greek Orthodox Christians follow
a different calendar which consists of
nearly 150 different fasting holidays.
Roman Catholics pay homage to the 40
days they believe Jesus fasted in the
desert by signifying the fasting of Lent.
That ritual has changed to only
abstaining from one thing, and it doesn't
even have to be food or water, but its

historical roots are still entwined with fasting. The Islamic calendar is probably one of the most well-known representations of fasting due to their annual month of Ramadan which is the 9th month of their calendar. During this month, believers fast from morning to night, for 30 days. This fasting is a bit different because they cannot even consume water, so many exceptions are made to people who have health issues, take medication throughout the day, or are pregnant or breastfeeding. Despite fasting from sunrise to sunset, it is important to note that due to this being a festival or celebratory month, studies have shown that caloric intake for Muslims actually increases during the month due to eating more fatty or fried foods.

The Jewish calendar also has nearly 25 days where Jews are encouraged to fast. Much like Muslims, their fasts also begin from sunrise and end when they see the first stars in the sky. Yom Kippur is one of the most popular fasting holidays with nearly a 25-hour-long fast, which signifies the "Day of Atonement." It's considered one of the holiest days in the Jewish religion where believers can fast to repent for the sins they've committed the previous year. Buddhist monks also undergo rituals of fasting and often have days where they only drink water to undergo spiritual cleansing. Hinduism also has many observances of fasting depending on the ascending and descending of the moon.

As we briefly mentioned above, with many of these world religions, there are exceptions given when it comes to individuals and their physical health. People are who have a severe illness where they take medicine or insulin throughout the day, who are not physically strong enough, or require extra calories because they are pregnant, or breastfeeding are excused from fasting. Before deciding to implement a ritual of fasting in your routine, it's important you speak to your doctor to ensure you are able to go for a prolonged window without food and have no health risks.

## › RECAP

History has proven that our ancestors practiced fasting as a way to survive and flourish in their tribe when times of famine would occur. Great thinkers, philosophers, and even the first well-known doctors recommended fasting to their patients. Many world religions include fasting in their rituals, but they also have exceptions for patients who are ill and cannot partake in it. Fasting is a very achievable goal that you can do too!

# Chapter 2

# Who Should & Should Not Fast

When it comes to fasting, it's all about having the correct intention for it. If you are someone who is willing to put in the work and make lifestyle adjustments, then this book and fasting is a great method for you to try! Some people feel like they have reached a plateau of their weight loss or are unable to sustain whatever diet they're trying for any longer. If you are someone who understands the historical context of fasting and how society has changed to where we consume so many calories in a short amount of time, you could be someone who adjusts to fasting and can see the health benefits associated with it.

So, what the categories of people who should partake in fasting if they and

their doctors have determined they are
physically able to?

## Healthy Adults

If you are a healthy adult without the need to take medication throughout the day or with health concerns, then it's perfectly healthy for you to fast from time to time. In fact, if you feel you're having trouble losing weight and are willing to make the sacrifice of going for a block of time without food, then you can try fasting!

## Adults With Signs Of Insulin Resistance

Insulin resistance occurs when your cells start becoming insensitive to insulin in the bloodstream which forces the body to produce glucose. This can mean a high level of glucose in the bloodstream and unstable blood sugar levels which can lead to Type 2 diabetes. Studies have shown that fasting can help lower these levels and allow the cells to become better at reading insulin levels.

## Adults Struggling To Lose Weight

If you have tried all the diets and made healthy lifestyle choices but are still struggling to lose weight and reach your health goals, fasting could be something you try. Especially if you feel you are having trouble containing the calories you eat and maybe going "cold turkey" and avoiding food for longer blocks of time could be the discipline you need. Fasting is a great method for many people who have reached a weight loss plateau but need a change in their routine in order to see results.

## Adults Looking To Improve Their Overall Health

If you're looking to improve your health more than just losing some pounds, fasting is the perfect answer for you. You gain mental acuity, better focus and concentration, and improved body composition and body mass index results. Along with these benefits, you could prevent or improve several health conditions like high blood pressure, high blood sugar levels, or high cholesterol.

## Adults Who Want To Take Charge Of Their Caloric Intake

Do you sometimes feel like you're overeating throughout the day? That you have too many snacks between meals? Is that affecting your health, your concentration, and your weight? One of the great ways to "cut yourself off" from calories is to extend your fasting window time. Giving yourself 12 hours or 18 hours when you do not eat is a great way to remind yourself to enjoy the food you do eat. For many people, fasting is a great way to do that with the bonus of improving their health!

What types of people are not our target audience for this book?

# Children

Most children who are under the age of 18 should not be fasting or going without food for extended periods of time. That's because the window of puberty is very important and requires a healthy diet of vitamins, minerals, and varieties of food for growing children and teenagers. The exception to this may be obese or overweight children struggling with their weight, but even then, you should go through other steps to restructure their diet, cut junk food and eat healthily, and implement a routine of exercise.

## Pregnant Or Breastfeeding Women

Exact research regarding how fasting affects women in this condition is still unsure, but most doctors would agree that extra calories are required. In fact, with most pregnancies, a moderate weight gain of 15 to 25 pounds is recommended. If exclusively breastfeeding, extra calories are also required to produce milk. Women in this stage of life should avoid fasting until they no longer require the extra calories.

## Vegans And Vegetarians

This book talks about the carnivore diet which is focused on eating meat and fish along with dairy and eggs. With a diet focused on fatty meats and healthy proteins, vegans and vegetarians aren't going to be able to follow. But intermittent fasting by itself is still something they could accommodate into their diet if they choose to!

## People With Underlying Medical Conditions Or Who Take Prescription Medication

If you have a severe medical condition that requires frequent medication throughout the day, or even a condition like diabetes, heart disease, or autoimmune disorders, you should avoid fasting and speak to your doctor before making any changes in your dietary routine. Chances are that with your medical requirements and need for medication, fasting is not going to be viable for you. People who have a history with eating disorders or body dysmorphia issues should abstain from fasting and speak to their doctor or therapist about any body issues they are feeling.

## People Who Want A Magical Fix To Their Weight Problems

If you're looking for a quick and painless way to lose weight, then this book and fasting probably aren't for you. Fasting takes time and purpose, as well as a mental and physical concentration on your goal. That means you have to be steadfast and be willing to put in the work to see your results. If you don't want to do the work, then this method isn't for you!

## People Who Aren't Open-minded

If you aren't willing to make a sacrifice then fasting may not be something you're willing to do. Giving up something is hard - giving up food may be even harder! You have to be willing to see the end results and make that sacrifice in the present day. If that's not something you're willing to do or to get out of your comfort zone, then

fasting might not be the right method
for you.

## › RECAP

---

Your health is first and foremost important so you should talk to your doctor before implementing a routine of fasting. If you are a healthy adult without medical limitations, then fasting could be great for you, especially if you want to improve your health and are willing to take on a challenge to do it! If you have a medical condition, take prescription medication, have a history with eating disorders, are pregnant or breastfeeding, or still a child, then fasting may not be for you.

## › ACTION ITEMS

---

Check with your doctor to see if fasting is right for you.

# Chapter 3

# The Benefits Of Fasting

Fasting has been shown to have many health benefits with scientific studies that lay out the evidence. It can seem counterintuitive that going without food can actually improve your health, but it can reverse many ongoing symptoms or even prevent future ones!

What are some benefits of fasting that may convince you to take part in it?

## Aids Weight Loss

Obviously, the first benefit of fasting we will mention is that it can help you lose weight effectively. When you are fasting, you are reducing your overall caloric intake which can actually boost your metabolism. That means you not only lose the weight, but you're more likely to keep it off! Studies have found that intermittent fasting can decrease body weight and weight loss up to 10 over a span of mere weeks! That means you're not only losing weight, but also losing excess fat you have stored away because when fasting, the body is more likely to burn fat reserves. You're losing fat instead of muscle tissue which means you can still build muscle and keep a toned body.

## Reduces Insulin Resistance

For people who are at risk of diabetes or have diabetes in their family, many studies have found that fasting can improve blood sugar control and significantly decrease blood sugar levels. When the body begins to lose its sensitivity to insulin, it's unable to transport glucose molecules from your bloodstream to your cells. That means the glucose stays in the blood and raises your blood sugar which causes more insulin to be produced. Fasting has been shown to reduce the resistance the cells have towards insulin which will prevent blood sugar spikes and crashes in your sugar levels.

## Fights Inflammation

Though normal flares of inflammation are common as we age, it's chronic inflammation that can be very dangerous to the body. It can lead to an umbrella of diseases such as cancer, heart disease, and arthritis. The good news is that studies have found fasting can decrease the levels of inflammation in the body and hopefully prevent these diseases. A study found that adults who fasted intermittently for one fast had decreased levels of inflammatory markers after they were tested. Two more studies conducted on mice found that following a diet that had a very low caloric intake to mimic fasting could help treat certain chronic inflammatory conditions like multiple sclerosis. This is great news for people who suffer from the early onset of these diseases but feel healthy enough to fast to combat these symptoms.

## Can Improve Heart Health

Believe it or not, fasting has been shown to improve many signs of cardiovascular disease such as lowering levels of fatty triglycerides in the blood, high cholesterol levels and decreasing blood pressure. Considering that heart disease accounts for more than 30% of deaths in the world, many people who have early warning signs would love to find something to reverse high symptoms that prove effective. A study following more than 100 obese adults found that intermittent fasting done over 3 weeks improved many high-risk heart disease signs such as high blood pressure, total cholesterol and "bad" LDL cholesterol numbers. With fasting also significantly lowering your risk of diabetes, that's a great sign since diabetes can be a major risk factor for heart disease.

## Increases Secretion Of Human Growth Hormone (HGH)

HGH is a protein that is important for many aspects of our growth including weight loss, metabolism, and muscle strength. The body naturally secretes large amounts of HGH during puberty in the teenage years, but the secretion slows into adulthood. Studies have shown that fasting can naturally increase HGH levels in adults. This is good news for weightlifters or bodybuilders who are in the department of growing muscle and wish to do so naturally instead of using outlawed products. Implementing a routine of fasting could help you do that!

# Cancer Treatment

Most of the research regarding the effects of fasting and cancer have been done in animals and cells solely in laboratories, so it's still unsure of how the human body would respond. But there have been promising studies in mice that show fasting could block tumor formation and even increase the effectiveness of chemotherapy drugs.

## Improves Brain Function And
## Mental Acuity

Many studies have found that fasting can have a positive effect on brain health and increase the number of nerve cells that enhance cognitive function. That means better brain functioning shown through longer attention span, more focus, and clear mental acuity. Scientists theorize that after a large meal, the body tends to use the food and go into overdrive at the sudden surge of glucose and carbohydrates. Overactivity is not necessarily a bad thing, but it can distract the brain from focusing on one task at a time. When fasting, the brain goes into "survival mode" and conserves its energy to one focus which can significantly improve brain power.

## Protects Against Neurodegenerative Diseases Like Alzheimer's And Parkinson's

With this improved mental functioning and the protection of nerve cells from degeneration, the body can clean out damaged nerve cells and generate new ones for better mental functioning. This is a great sign and can prevent the body from neurodegenerative diseases that can greatly impact the mind and mental functioning.

## Improves Mood

It seems counteractive to think that going without food can improve your mood! But the truth is, many studies have found that fasting for a period of time can actually improve your mood and help with mental disorders like depression or anxiety. The more carbohydrate-loaded food you eat and the more frequent snacks you have will cause your body's sugar levels to spike. Too many spikes can confuse the body and cause it to enter stress mode and release cortisol, the body's stress hormone, to stabilize blood sugar levels. When you are not eating, the body doesn't experience these spikes and can harness energy from fat reserves you already have stored.

**Keeps Cells Young And Healthy**

Fasting can improve the lifespan of your cells and slow the aging of the mitochondrial networks in the center of them. Mitochondria are the cellular part that generates power for your cells. When cells start to age, these mitochondria become weak and defective. But a 2017 study at Harvard found that fasting can keep mitochondria strong and able to continue process energy which is critical to keep your cells healthy for a longer period of time.

## Strengthens The Immune System

Fasting actually lowers your white blood cell count which triggers the body to regenerate those cells and produce new immune system cells. This process is called "autophagy," or the body's biological method of disposing of damaged or old cells and creating new, energetic ones. A study at the University of South California found that fasting anywhere from 2 to 4 days can actually regenerate a person's immune system and promote stem-based cells. With a "newer" immune system, a person has a lower risk of neurological diseases and fight off viruses and bacteria.

## It's Easy To Follow!

Unlike other complicated diets or exercise lifestyles, fasting is very easy and simple to follow for beginners. What are you eating? Nothing! Instead of worrying about buying the right ingredients, planning a complicated meal, or ensuring you are counting calories of everything you're eating, fasting is very simple because you're cutting the headache of food out of your diet. Instead, you focus on eating healthy when you are not fasting and implementing a healthy routine of exercise to further improve your health. The ease of fasting is what appeals to many people who don't have the time to count macros or spend money on fancy ingredients.

## Improves Eating Patterns

Many people have an unhealthy relationship with food - not that they're eating too little, but that they are eating too much. We often take food for granted simply because it's always around us and easily available to us. Whether it's a full pantry at home, the drive-thru near work, or the vending machine in the lobby, many of us are always filling our hour with some snack or another. With fasting, you can find a correct eating pattern that works for you that does not involve overeating. Instead, you can build a routine that works for your body and promotes overall health for your future. Fasting allows you to dedicate time for your meals so you can really enjoy them and not feel guilty for eating too much or binging on extra calories throughout the day.

## › RECAP

The research is astounding when it comes to what fasting can do. From lowering your blood pressure to stabilizing your blood sugar levels, to reducing the risk of Alzheimer's and Parkinson's disease to strengthening your immune system, fasting is something that can improve the health of many people. The way that it is so easy to follow makes it very appealing to people who don't want to meal plan or count calories!

## › ACTION ITEMS

Research what would be your motivation for fasting and how it could improve your individual health.

# Chapter 4

# The Science Behind Fasting

As we read the benefits of fasting and how it can improve your overall health, it's also important to be aware of the science behind fasting and how these benefits occur in our body.

Calorie restriction is a very important goal of fasting. It's reducing the average daily intake of calories to what you would normally have had but without depriving yourself of nutrition or essential vitamins and minerals that are also necessary to the body. So, for example, whatever block of time a fasting person is abstaining from food, it's important that they still have a balanced and healthy diet when they are allowed to eat. That might mean fewer calories because you have shortened the window of time to eat, but it still means eating healthy and ensuring you remain in good health.

Restricting calories has to be a consistent pattern over a period of time. If anything, we're often eating too many calories that we don't need! Many doctors and researchers believe that following a rotating fasting routine, such as the 5:2 routine, can put your body through a helpful kind of "therapy" to wean off the extra calories. Total fasting diets are a bad idea because they cause you to lose muscle mass. But with following a pattern of fasting, and then eating days, people will consume fewer calories which will help them lose excess weight in fat, not in muscle. Not only that, studies show that it can increase your metabolism overall which means that even if you stop fasting, you should still be able to consume fewer calories and feel full for longer.

A lot of research has been conducted on calorie restriction on lab animals to get an idea of how this would apply to humans. Studies have found that with rats or mice were given anywhere from 10% to 40% fewer calories, they were able to live longer lifespans than other counterparts and showed reduced rates of diseases. Despite the lower caloric intake, they were still given the essential nutrients and were not deprived. Another long-term study on monkeys found that monkeys who ate 30% fewer calories than their counterparts had a lower risk of diseases and lived longer. More research needs to be conducted on humans in order to understand how reducing caloric intake would help us overall. Studies have shown that individuals on a lower calorie diet tend to have less risk for diabetes and heart disease, which is a promising sign that less really is more when it comes to food and caloric intake.

Insulin sensitivity is another important topic related to fasting. When we eat a meal, the body digests this food into glucose molecules for energy and works to transport it through the bloodstream to your cells. Insulin is a hormone which the pancreas produces after a meal so the cells can begin to absorb glucose and fuel themselves. If your body is losing sensitivity to insulin, that means the cells are unable to respond to the insulin signals and do not intake those glucose molecules. The glucose stays in your bloodstream, and it becomes stored as excess fat. Meanwhile, your body continues to produce insulin because the cells haven't received the signal!

When this communication in the body is broken down, insulin resistance occurs, and those glucose molecules do not get processed. Sometimes, the pancreas can produce more insulin, and that gets your cells working, but insulin sensitivity is what occurs when the cells are irresponsible to the flood of insulin in the bloodstream. The problem is because the pancreas has to produce a lot of insulin, which makes it unable to work properly. That's the underlying symptom of insulin deficiency which can lead to diabetes.

Often many people have insulin resistance and have no idea for years. Unless there's a family history of diabetes where people are on alert for warning signs, other people could simply have the symptoms without realizing it. Some of these symptoms include fatigue, patches of dark skin, extra weight you just can't lose, acne, polycystic ovarian syndrome or PCOS in women, cravings after mealtimes, fluid retention, and high blood pressure. With these symptoms so varied, it can be hard to diagnose insulin resistance.

Thankfully, research has shown that fasting is a great way to increase your body's sensitivity to insulin. That's because when you are fasting, the body decreases its reliance on glucose as a source of energy and focuses on ketones instead. These ketones are made from the extra fat molecules you already have stored. With these ketones being produced, the body shifts into a state called "ketosis," which is great because insulin doesn't have to be produced! This means your pancreas can rest and recover from false flares of having to produce more insulin for the body. With better insulin sensitivity, you actually can eat less because the body has gotten better at delivering all the nutrients available to the cells. You do not have to overcompensate and eat more which means you're reducing your caloric intake and can lose weight!

When you are eating meals, the glucose produced from food can cause blood sugar spikes. But with fasting as a part of your routine, the body produces ketones instead. These will not cause blood sugar levels to rise like glucose does since it is a simple sugar molecule. Ketones are produced from fat, so they do not affect the blood sugar the same way. They give the body a rich source of energy which can actually improve mental clarity and attention span.

We talked about fasting also stimulating the cellular process of autophagy. Autophagy comes from the Greek words "auto," meaning self, and "phagein," which means to eat. This cellular process was discovered in the 1960s when researchers began to notice cells were destroying their parts and "eating" them or taking them into their own cellular body. In fact, in 2016, Japanese scientist Yoshinori Ohsumi was awarded the Nobel Prize in Physiology or Medicine for his study in autophagy of yeast and how essential genes were necessary for cells to be capable of autophagy.

This function is crucial for the immune system where old cellular parts are broken down to develop new cells that will become a part of the immune system. Mitophagy is a part of autophagy where the body specifically takes in damaged mitochondria cellular parts and uses them to produce stronger and more resilient mitochondria.

Think of autophagy as a "cleansing" of the system and checking which cells are still performing at a high level and which have become older or slower. The better our cells perform, the healthier we will be! Our immune systems will be stronger, our brains will work faster, and our bodies will be more resistant to wear and tear that comes with aging. This process is essential for our health!

## › RECAP

The science behind fasting shows how it takes place from making your body more sensitive to insulin to stabilize your blood sugar levels without frequent blood spikes due to carbohydrates in your diet. It's not only that, fasting allows your body to stop relying on glucose for energy and to use the process of ketosis instead. This is what helps you burn off the excess weight!

# Chapter 5

# Fasting & Autophagy

Autophagy is like the body's system of cleaning house. That's when our cells begin to look at other cells and see if they have any weaknesses and are not functioning up to a certain level. If they have damaged parts or are worn out, the cell will immerse itself around the weaker cell for energy or for cellular parts. Many researchers describe it as a recycling program! It's a biological system that allows our cells to become more efficient by getting rid of damaged or weaker counterparts. These damaged cells can be quite dangerous in the long run because they could contain cancer or create a cascading effect of neurodegenerative diseases like Parkinson's or Alzheimer's.

Autophagy actually occurs in the body as a response to stress. So if you want to rev up your body's "recycling system," and ensure you're getting rid of those older cells, then you do have to put your body through some sort of stress in order to initiate autophagy.

What are the main ways to trigger autophagy and boost your immune system?

## Exercise

Exercise is one of the most popular ways for people to unknowingly begin the process of autophagy in their cells. Exercise puts stress on the body! When you're working out, sweating, and you're feeling that burn from your workout, your muscles are stretching and creating microscopic tears. When this happens, the body quickly rushes to heal and become stronger in case you go through that routine again. That's how your muscle mass increases. Studies had

found in mice that when they went
through physical exercise on a treadmill,
the rate of their cells going through
autophagy drastically increased. The
more exercise they went through, the
higher the rate of cellular autophagy.
With humans, the exact level of exercise
is still undetermined, and it's hard to
answer that question with a specific time
or exercise routine. That's because so
many factors play a role in exercising
such as individual body mass, body type,
and physical activity level. But you can
probably assume that after an intense
workout, your body is getting the
benefits of autophagy and able to start
the biological process under the stress
you've produced.

# Lower Carb Intake

As we mentioned in the previous section, lowering your carbohydrate intake begins a process in the body called "ketosis." With ketosis, the body uses fat you have stored to create ketone molecules for energy. Following this diet has many health benefits and is often followed by bodybuilders or weightlifters who are looking to shed extra fat. Ketosis has also been shown to initiate autophagy in the body because of the metabolic change it starts. You can get the benefits of the added stress to your body without needing to fast or go without food - you're simply changing what you're eating. The keto diet can be very specific though and requires counting your daily macro intake to ensure you're consuming around 70% high-quality fats, 20% protein, and 5% carbohydrates. It can be tough for some people considering that carbohydrates make up nearly three-fourths of our daily diet! But it is a way to "shock" your body into changing the way it harnesses energy which will successfully begin autophagy for your cells.

# Fasting

Eating or drinking like normal actually works against autophagy in the body. That's because the body's biological needs are being met and there's no stressful environment for it to adjust to. But when you fast for a period of time, the body sees it as a stressful act which it ultimately benefits from. Besides all the other health benefits we mentioned regarding fasting, it also promotes autophagy in the brain. This is very essential for keeping neural cells active and working at the highest functioning they can. A higher rate of autophagy in the brain can lower the risk of neurodegenerative diseases. Not only that, lab studies conducted on rodents found that intermittent fasting even improved brain structure, cognitive function, and neuroplasticity. Without similar studies conducted on humans, it's unclear whether this is linked to autophagy, but a lot of research on autophagy has shown how important it is in neural activity.

Though all of these scenarios of stress that the body can experience, most scientists believe that in an anthropological sense, fasting is the most natural one for the human species. That's because our ancestors dealt with times of feast and famine when they were first in their hunter and gatherer tribes. Humans had no choice but to adjust to environmental conditions and man-made conditions like wartime when food would be scarce. It was only much later that humans put a positive spin on dieting or exercising. For our early ancestors, being able to endure periods of time without food was a quality that ensured their survival and actually increased their eventual lifespan. Adjustment is a natural part of our body's creation, and there is always a "back up plan" if you are fasting or going without food for an extended period of time. In this case, fasting allows your body to use reserves already stored away instead of relying on the continuous flow of calories you're eating throughout the day.

It's important to note that autophagy is a natural process that occurs in the body. It's how your cell "recycles" older cells to create new ones. Cells consist of cytoplasm and cellular parts. In autophagy, the cell parts and the cytoplasm fluid are removed and recycled to the newer cell. This is good news because research has shown that there are many disorders that are linked to abnormal functioning of autophagy in the body. If a cell is not properly "recycled" or its dysfunctional cellular parts are left functioning, it could cause devastating health conditions. Autophagy-related genes were first identified in the 1990s and further highlighted how important the process of autophagy is for the body.

Some of these disorders that are considered autophagy-related genes include: Parkinson's disease, Crohn's Disease, Vici Syndrome, and types of cancer. Cancer is different because it is not necessarily genetically-related, but researchers have found that if autophagy is not working correctly in the body, the tumor will stay established and the cells keep it from being destroyed as your body fights cancer.

When we see what could go wrong if autophagy is not working, we can understand why people want to go through efforts to add stress to their body to initiate this biological reaction! This is the body's natural way of ensuring the balance between healthy and unhealthy cells and to hopefully prevent the risk of several neurodegenerative diseases and cancer. It decreases the oxidative stress on the body to keep the cells younger and healthier and increases the elimination of waste to prevent mutations that could occur. Ultimately, the goal of autophagy is to keep you as healthy as possible and increase your lifespan.

## › RECAP

Autophagy is a biological process that occurs to "recycle" older or damaged cells to keep the body's cellular system working at top efficiency. Higher rates of this "clean up" is linked to lower rates of neurodegenerative diseases. With this information, it's only natural to want to keep our bodies healthy and young. To do that, you must exert stress on the body which involves situations like exercise and fasting.

# Chapter 6

# The Carnivore Diet & Fasting

The carnivore diet has become one of the most talked about diets in nutrition trends because of how its main principle is to encourage people to eat meat. It's a bit controversial for that exact reason because we've heard for so long how too much meat can create diseases and clog your arteries and how moderation is key. But with this diet comes unexpected health benefits such as weight loss and better mental acuity, so it's worth looking at.

This diet is one that encourages its followers to eat only animal foods and stay away from the rest. That means you are severely limiting your intake of carbohydrates and plant-based foods. Think of it as the complete opposite of the vegan diet! A lot like the ketogenic diet, the carnivore diet also relies heavily on fats and proteins as the main component of fuel. Just like the ketogenic diet, the carnivore diet is also chosen because of its health benefits which are very similar to keto. It's very appealing to people who don't want to remember lists of ingredients they should and should not eat because the rule is very simple - animal foods are allowed!

So what are you allowed to eat and what should you avoid? Let's go over the lists now.

# *Foods You Should Eat On The Carnivore Diet*

## Meat

---

Red meat is going to be the tenet of this diet. This is going to be where the majority of your calories come from throughout the day since you are not going to be eating carbohydrates or consuming fruits or vegetables. In other words, the majority of your meals will consist of a lot of fatty cuts of steak!

## Fish

---

Fish is another rich source of protein you can have in your diet. The fattier the fish is, the better which includes types like halibut and salmon. This is a great way to add some variety to your meals, so you are getting healthy omega 3 fatty acids and a change from the red meat.

# Dairy

Since dairy technically comes from animals like butter, cheese, and milk, these are allowed on the carnivore diet. That means you don't have to make the substitutions as you usually would on a keto diet. You can continue to have a diet full of your dairy favorites.

## Animal Fat Products

These are products like lard or ghee and other animal-derived fats that you are encouraged to continue eating on the carnivore diet.

Now that we've discussed foods that you should eat, let's talk about the foods you should avoid.

# Foods To Avoid On The Carnivore Diet

### Carbohydrates

---

Whether it's bread, vegetables, or artificial candy, you want to stay away from carbohydrates because they are not allowed on the carnivore diet.

### Supplements

---

Any other sort of supplements should be avoided. The idea is that your body is going to derive all the necessary nutrients it needs just from the animal products.

## More About The Carnivore Diet

The idea of the carnivore diet originates from the idea that the human population has never lived in a time where eating such a heavily plant-based diet was followed. But there have many of our ancestral tribes that have followed mostly an animal-based diet like the Nomads of Mongolia, the Canadian Inuits who ate mostly fish, and the Masai from East Africa who consumed mostly meat and dairy. The consumption of animal products was considered a high mark of strength in these cultures.

The idea of this diet is very similar to the keto diet where your intake will consist of protein and fat sources. When the body no longer relies on simple carbohydrates for energy, it will enter the state of ketosis where it uses fats to produce ketones for a richer source of energy. These can improve mental focus and give you an extra boost of energy! That's also how you're able to shed the extra weight you haven't been able to get rid of. The two diets are similar, but the carnivore diet goes one step further and is considered more restrictive regarding the intake of carbohydrates. The keto diet still encourages some low-carb foods like vegetables, coconut oil, nuts, and fruit. The carnivore diet also does not have macronutrient ratios to follow like keto is firm about. With you removing carbohydrates from your diet, you will surely reach ketosis as opposed to keto where you have to maintain less than ~5% carbohydrates to ensure the same process takes place.

So now that you have a basic understanding of the carnivore diet, let's discuss the benefits you'll get by following it.

# Benefits Of The Carnivore Diet

As we mentioned above, the benefits of the carnivore diet are very similar to the keto diet since both require primarily eating fat and protein. Remember, the carnivore goes a step further and cuts out all carbohydrates! There are some great benefits to this diet that include:

## Improves The Body's Digestive System

Contrary to what we've been told, researchers of the carnivore diet believe that cutting fiber from your diet can help your digestive system especially if you have flares of diarrhea or constipation. A gastroenterology study has shown that patients with less fiber showed a great improvement in their digestive issues like bloating, gassiness, and cramps. This theory supports the idea that it's the variance amount of fiber in our diet that is often causing our digestive issues. By cutting it out completely on the carnivore diet, you could be helping your digestive system.

## Better mental clarity

With the carnivore diet, the body will now be harvesting ketones for energy instead of glucose molecules. Glucose is a simple sugar which is quickly burned and considered a "quick and cheap" energy fuel. Ketone consists of high-quality fats and allows you to feel an increase in mental clarity, focus, and attention. Studies have shown that people on a diet that follows ketosis have better mental recollection and memory recall, as well as an improvement in their mood! With simple carbohydrates, the body quickly burns up this fuel and then needs more which leaves you with blood sugar spikes.

## Faster Weight Loss

When it comes down to it, the carnivore diet is a great way to help you lose stubborn weight you haven't been able to get rid of. If your body isn't insulin sensitive, the problem could be that carbohydrates are being stored as fat instead of energy. By completely cutting carbohydrates from your diet, you're changing the way your body uses its food and allowing it to go through ketosis instead. This means maintaining and burning through your stored fat reserves and getting rid of that weight!

## Adjusts Hormone Imbalances

Studies have shown that diets such as the keto and carnivore one have been shown to improve hormone imbalances that occur. That's because sex hormones like estrogen and testosterone are composed mainly of fat and protein molecules like lipids and amino acids. What does the carnivore diet consist of? Fat and protein! For people who suffer from hormone imbalances, especially women who may have PCOS or irregular menstrual cycles, the carnivore diet could adjust their hormone levels back to normal.

## It's Super Easy To Follow!

The carnivore diet appeals to so many people who want to lose the weight and see the health benefits without worrying about counting calories, meal prepping and special recipes, or keeping track of daily

78

macronutrients. It's so very simple! If it's an animal-derived product, you can eat it! If it's carbohydrates, you can't! This simplicity allows people a lot of flexibility with their schedule and their lifestyle and makes it very easy to keep up with the diet even when eating out. The simpler it is, the more likely you are to continue following it and see the benefits through!

Now that you understand the benefits of the carnivore diet, let's discuss

## *Fasting with the Carnivore Diet*

As we mentioned above, the carnivore diet has many health benefits that can be achieved without fasting. But as we've elaborated in this book, fasting also has many health benefits. By fasting on the carnivore diet, you have the opportunity to greatly enhance your health and gain many overall benefits. Even if it's just a 12-hour fast after dinner, you're still gaining the many health benefits we mentioned and allowing your body to shed excess weight. It's allowing you to benefit from two things!

The reason why many find the carnivore diet a great complement with intermittent fasting routines is because the diet is so rich in protein and fat. That means you're able to have a filling, satisfying meal that gives you the energy you need to make it through your fasting period. As opposed to a diet high in carbohydrates where the glucose fuel is quickly burned, this diet is harvesting energy from ketones which are formed from the healthy fats you are eating. That means more energy to get you through your fasting period so that you don't feel hungry or deal with cravings. Think about it - you feel full for a lot longer after having a steak with butter than a vegetable-loaded salad!

What are some different types of fasts you can follow on the carnivore diet? Here are some popular intermittent fasting routines you can follow:

## 12/12 Method

This is the most popular method where you fast for 12 hours. You might be nearly doing it without even realizing it! The most common way this is done is not to eat after dinnertime and ensure you're maintaining a 12-hour window until you eat in the morning. For example, if you are done with dinner by 7:30 PM, ensure you don't eat again until 7:30 AM the next morning.

## 16/8 Method

This method involves fasting for about 16 hours for men, and 14-15 hours for women since women tend to have a lower body mass index. You can have an 8 to 10-hour "eating window" where you can fit 2-3 meals and load up on fats and proteins. For example, let's say you have your dinner at 8 PM. If you don't eat breakfast until 12 noon the next day, then you have fasted for 16 hours. For women, you could do slightly shorter fasts. If you're someone who already skips breakfast in the morning, this fasting method could work for you!

## 5:2 Diet

This is another popular fasting method where you would eat normally for 5 days of the week following your carnivore diet, and restrict calories on 2 days of the week. On the fasting days, it's recommended that men consume around 600 calories, and women consume 500 calories. You could follow this method by eating normally every day of the week except Mondays and Thursdays where you fast and ensure your small meals don't go over the caloric limit.

## Eat-Stop Eat

This is a method which involves completing a 24-hour fasting period once or twice a week. It can be tough and not for beginners! So, if you have dinner on Monday night at 7 PM, you will not eat another meal until the next night at 7 PM. That's completing a 24-hour period. You can do from breakfast to breakfast, or dinner to dinner, it depends on your preference. You can, of course, have non-caloric beverages and stay hydrated, but no solid food while fasting.

## › RECAP

---

The carnivore diet is a great supplement to fasting to ensure you are gaining all the health benefits you can. With this diet, you are cutting carbohydrates from your diet to ensure that your body will follow the path of ketosis to burn fat instead. By adding fasting to this diet, you're gaining the health benefits of those as well! There many fasting plans you can follow and fit around your busy lifestyle.

## › ACTION ITEMS

---

Plan a shopping list of carnivore diet foods to help you get even healthier. Plan which fasting method could work for your lifestyle.

# Chapter 7

# The Details of Fasting & How to Start

It can be intimidating when you first begin fasting, so it's important that you are aware of the "rules" and exactly what you are getting into! Many religions have different rituals of how they begin and end fasting periods, but for fasting on a carnivore diet, it's important you know what breaks a fast and when to avoid fasting.

First and foremost, you do want to check with your doctor to ensure that you have no health risks that would impede a fasting period. If you take medication or insulin throughout the day or have a severe medical condition, fasting may not be a viable option for you as opposed to someone who is pre-diabetic and battling the occasional high blood sugar level. You want to ensure you have the "all clear" from your doctor. Know that if you are feeling sick, you should stop at any time and assess your physical needs.

Next, you want to adjust your mindset of how you approach fasting. If you see it as "starving yourself" or a period of time you dread and see negatively, then your body and your mental state will reflect that. Instead, remind yourself that you are lucky enough to choose to fast. You know there is a meal waiting for you! You're just choosing not to eat it. You can start and stop anytime you want, and this is a purely voluntary decision that you are embarking on. You're making this choice for your health and because of the benefits that you have researched on and learned about. You want to gain those benefits too! This allows you to have a positive aspect about your fasting time and not see it as a struggling period you have to make it through.

Remind yourself of your "why" reason. Why is this important to you and why are you making this sacrifice? Are you hoping to lose weight you haven't been able to get rid of? Are you insulin resistant and you want to see if this makes changes in your blood sugar? Are you pre-diabetic and you want to stabilize your blood sugar levels in hopes of avoiding medication? Do you want to lower your blood pressure by your next check-up? Do you simply want to gain the benefits of longevity and hopefully prevent any debilitating diseases? The more strongly you feel about your goal, the more likely you will be to achieve it!

The fasting rules are very simple! Fasting is ideal for many people because there are no lists to memorize about what you can and cannot eat. Fasting, in this case, is defined as consuming only water, black coffee, or tea. You cannot have food or beverages that contain calories. You want to be sure that your tea and coffee do not contain sugar or creamer because those count as caloric intake. Following this very short list makes it very simple to know what you can and cannot have.

Your fast breaks if you unknowingly or willingly have food. When that happens, it's up to you how to proceed. If you obviously are not feeling well and need to break your fast, then you should take care of your health and do what your body needs. If you feel you can ignore that mouthful of food you had and continue with your fast, you can proceed. Forgive yourself and move on! You can pick up where you left off or start again on a new day - it's up to you to do what you need to get back on track.

You should try to avoid fasting in periods of stress. Whether that's a physical environment causing you stress or emotional toll, it may not be best for you to fast during a turbulent time in your life. Be sure you have the mindset and can avoid stress to focus on fasting and to remind yourself of the positive reasons you're taking part in it.

## *How to Start Fasting*

### Eliminate Snacks

If you want to ease your way into fasting, cutting snacks from your diet is a great way to start. Often we have food with us and eat it simply for the sake of something to do. Whether that's a granola bar in the car or something from the vending machine to munch on during a meeting, avoid those snacks and those extra calories which you will not need if you have healthy and filling meals.

### Set A Schedule

Even if you plan on fasting 12 hours or 16 hours, there's no schedule set for you. As long as you are sure to complete that time period, you can set the clock as you wish. If you prefer to eat dinner a little later like 8 PM then eat breakfast at 8 AM, you can do that. If you prefer an earlier meal so you can just have a cup of tea before bed, you could do 7 PM and then break your fast at 7 AM. The hour of the day depends on you! Adjust it to your schedule, so you feel most confident about your fasting.

## Stay Hydrated

Whether it's black coffee or unsweetened tea like we mentioned above, it's important that you are staying hydrated and especially that you are drinking enough water. These other beverages will act like a "filler" as you mimic the movements of drinking and filling your stomach. Caffeine actually helps dull hunger pangs so you can feel full for longer even on an empty stomach! You should always have water with you to ensure you are getting enough fluids. Sometimes, we feel like we are hungry, but we are actually thirsty instead!

## Stay Busy

One of the best tips when it comes to getting into the routine of fasting is filling your schedule! Most people find it easier to fast on a weekday because they will have work or school to keep them busy. That means less time to grab a meal or worry about how hungry you feel! So if you are trying to get through your 12- or 16-hour fasting window, be sure you have activities to keep you busy. Whether it's simply staying out of the house and away from food, maybe it's errands you've been meaning to run around town, or maybe you can go to the gym or take a walk around the block. The busier you feel, the less time you'll be agonizing about whether your fasting window is over.

## Eliminate Temptations

When you're watching TV, you're actually being bombarded with advertisements for food, snacks, restaurants, and many delicious things! Try to avoid those subliminal messages, and also stay away from places that are serving food. If you are hanging out with friends, see if you can hang out after mealtime, so there's no pressure for you to eat with them.

## Ease Into A Meal

---

When you are breaking your fast at the end of the fasting window, be as gentle as you can. A mistake many people make is having a large meal right when their time is up which can give you a stomach ache. It's nothing too serious, but it can be uncomfortable! So, go easy on yourself and maybe start with a small snack and then treat yourself to a delicious meal.

## Get Some Sleep

---

Sleep is going to be very important for you to maintain your energy and strength when you are fasting. Be sure you're getting a good night's sleep so that you wake up refreshed the next day. To put it simply, when you're sleeping, you're not hungry! So set up your day so that your sleep window can align with your fasting window. For example, if you have your

93

dinner at 7 PM, be sure to go to bed soon after so you aren't tempted for another snack. If you aren't breaking your fast until 8 AM, see if you can sleep as late as you can so that once you are up, you have just a little bit of time left in your fasting window. If you're going to skip dinner entirely, be sure you are keeping yourself busy and going to bed soon after.

## › RECAP

---

If you want to start fasting, it's important you first have a positive attitude and a goal in mind. Remind yourself what your reason is for fasting, whether it's losing weight, lowering your blood sugar level, or lowering your cholesterol or blood pressure. With your reason in mind, you can embark on fasting with these tips to help you gain success!

## › ACTION ITEMS

---

Find your motivation to fast and develop a positive attitude about it. Plan your fast and your meals and keep yourself busy and hydrated during your fasting period.

# Chapter 8

# Myths & Misconceptions About Fasting

With any new diet method becoming popular, there are going to be misconceptions and myths that you have to battle. With fasting, there tends to be a lot more criticism and negative perceptions simply because people consider it an extreme method. They don't know the history behind fasting or that it was something that came naturally to our ancestors. And people don't realize that the research shows the many health benefits of skipping a meal or two.

This section is all about debunking common myths about fasting so that you have the most accurate information as you add fasting to your routine.

# You Can't Survive Without Drinking Water

This is very true, and that's why fasting doesn't involve giving up water. In fact, be sure you drink enough water, have black coffee, and even unsweetened tea. Having some caffeine will actually help you when it comes to dulling your hunger pangs. You just want to be sure you're not adding cream or sugar because those contain calories. Staying hydrated is very important, and it's encouraged that you drink enough water. Be sure you have a water bottle with you at all times. Symptoms of dehydration can sneak up on you, especially if you are going through a long fast.

## Don't Ever Skip Breakfast

The idea that breakfast is the most important of the day has become a well-known saying, but it's not always true. Yes, eating breakfast in the morning tends to start your metabolism and quickly give you energy, but that's only because your cells are much more receptive to insulin after you slept all night and didn't eat anything. The body considers those 6 to 8 hours as a fasting window, and the next time you eat, it coincides as breakfast time. If you love breakfast and consider it an essential meal of your day, then don't skip it. Start your fast after that time and see if you can end it 12 or 16 hours later. You should adjust your fasting window to what works for you.

# Fasting Over 12 Hours Is Bad For You

That is true that when you see the number, it can seem very high. 12 hours, or 16 hours, it sounds like a long period of time to get through. But when you put 12 hours into perspective, you might be almost fasting for that long without realizing it. For example, let's say you have dinner every night around 7:30 or 8 PM, and only have a cup of nighttime tea before bed. Then, in the morning, maybe you're busy with morning routines and getting the kids to school that you have a large cup of coffee and don't get your first bite of breakfast until nearly 7 AM. That's nearly 12 hours right there! All fasting does is extend that window and make you responsible for avoiding food and anything with calories.

## Fasting Will Interfere With Athletic Performance

This is one of the big myths that stop people from fasting. They think that they will lose their drive and energy when it comes to training sessions or going to the gym. But studies show that fasting does not hinder your aerobic or anaerobic activity performances. When you begin fasting, you might feel slow or lethargic in the beginning. But that's the same when you start any new diet and make a change to your routine, whether that's quitting nicotine or quitting carbohydrates, or deciding to fast for a period of time. As we've explained, when you're fasting the body turns to its fat reserves to burn fuel by producing ketones. These actually give you a burst of energy and could improve your performance, not just physically, but also mentally.

## You'll Gain All The Weight Back Once You Stop Fasting

This is a common misconception that people like to say whenever you make a change in your diet or routine. The truth is, what happens after you stop fasting, or after you stop dieting, is up to you! You will gain back the weight if you return to your old habits and end up consuming additional calories to make up for those you lost when fasting. But if fasting has helped you take a step back from your reliance on food and quit eating more calories than you need, then you will continue to have a healthy relationship with food and hopefully keep off the weight you lost. It's up to you!

# Blood Sugar Will Drop

Research has shown that when you are fasting your blood sugar levels remain relatively stable (except if you have diabetes). In fact, when you're fasting, the body switches from using glucose as fuel to ketones which keep your blood sugars more stable. When you eat, your body actually releases a rush of insulin to stabilize your blood sugar levels. With fasting, you're not eating for a certain amount of time, which means that your body can stay responsive to insulin and keep your blood sugar stable. In fact, if you're craving food throughout the day, it's probably a sign that your blood sugar is too high instead of too low!

## Fasting Loses Muscle Gains

This is another myth that often scares people off fasting. The thing to remember is that when you eat, the digestion process is a long one. Even hours later, your body is still breaking down the proteins and carbohydrates you've eaten into fuel for energy. If you skip one meal, or two, it doesn't mean the body will turn on itself and eat away your muscle. In fact, research proves it will use its fat reserves first instead of turning to muscle! A lot of athletes incorporate fasting into their routine so they can get rid of excess fat. Fasting for 12 hours or 16 hours, or even 20, isn't enough time where the body will consume its own muscle mass. If you are an athlete and you're worried about this but still interested in fasting, talk to your trainer for advice and reassurance on how to begin!

# I Can't Survive Without Food

The human body is a medical marvel. If you think about it in a historical lens, our ancestors were made to survive many periods of uncertainty whether that was war, natural disasters, or famine and illness. When they had food, they ate, and when they didn't, they adjusted. It's the individuals who were able to withstand a little bit of hunger that were able to survive and flourish in their tribe. Of course, it's important to enjoy food and feel full, but it's also important to give your body a break and allow yourself the health benefits that come with fasting. If 24 hours seems too long for you, go shorter! Fasting is up to you and your comfort and routine. You can make it work for your lifestyle.

## So, Going Without Food Can Actually Improve My Health? Really?

Yes!

As we've explained in Chapter 3, there are many scientific studies that show how fasting can improve your health. Whether it's protecting you from neurodegenerative diseases or cancer or helping you lower your cholesterol and blood pressure, the research proves that you could extend your lifespan simply by making fasting a part of your life. Whether you're aiming just to lose weight or stabilize your blood sugar levels, fasting could be something you partake in to improve your health especially if you have a family history of diabetes or cardiovascular disease. The evidence is all there – it's up to you to make the change!

## › RECAP

---

Like many diets, fasting also some myths that surround it despite being untrue. You will not gain back the weight as long as you continue to have a healthy relationship with food, you can work out, you won't lose muscle mass, and you may even gain more energy and mental focus! With these misconceptions clarified, you can feel confident about including fasting in your life.

## › ACTION ITEM

---

Educate yourself on these misconceptions of fasting so that you can feel confident the next time you hear criticism about fasting.

# Chapter 9

# Helpful Tips & Tricks

If you're interested in more helpful tips and tricks for fasting, here are some things that could work for you!

## Stay Hydrated

Whether that's drinking water, or tea or coffee, ensure you continuously have those beverages nearby during your fasting window. Caffeine is actually great during your fast because it dulls the body's hunger and makes you feel fuller than you are. Have you noticed when you have a couple cups of coffee you forget about eating for a while? Remember to exclude things like creamer, milk, or sugar from your drinks because those do count as calories. Dehydration can sneak up on you, so it's important you are keeping track of your water intake.

## Incorporate Bone Broth

Bone broth is a very nutritious dish packed with vitamins, minerals, electrolytes, and water. It's very hydrating, so it's a great way to ensure you're still getting water in an alternate method. It's a traditional dish that's believed to have healing properties. You can add a good dash of salt to ensure you're having a balance of electrolytes as well (because you lose electrolytes after urinating). Find a delicious recipe and make it in batches, so you have it to consume.

## Exercise Reasonably

Most people who fast find that if they exercise before a meal, then they can eat right after their workout. If you eat after exercise, you might find yourself famished after your workout! Exercise is perfectly okay to do when fasting as long as you don't feel tired or weak. Most research has found that mild to moderate exercise performance, and training has not suffered for people who are fasting. Most dieters felt they reported more energetic when fasting! You don't have to run a marathon, but incorporating some yoga, walking, jogging, or biking can be a great way to burn restless energy and improve your health too!

## Be Selective With Your Support Team

Some people might start criticizing or berating you for fasting. In most circles, it's still considered an "extreme" method, despite the historical evidence and the many world religions that partake in fasting. If you feel judged or you feel uncomfortable when people bring up your fasting routine, don't mention it to them. Politely decline food when offered, or try to stay away from those gatherings at mealtimes. Fasting depends on your attitude so staying positive is very important. As long as you have done the research, know the health benefits, and know the safety concerns, stay positive about your goals and your journey!

## Find Ways To Relax

As we mentioned before, the busier you are, the faster it will seem like your fasting period is going and keep your mind off the temptation of food. Find a relaxing technique that works for you. Whether that's some yoga, guided meditation techniques, deep breathing, reading, or knitting... find something that can keep you busy and keep your mind off your fast (especially if the last few hours seem like they're dragging by). You don't want to expend too much energy if you feel tired, but keep your mind engaged and occupied.

## Don't Binge

Sometimes people make the mistake of eating too much after their fast has ended because they feel like they are starving. But if you're simply consuming all those calories you missed out on, then you're not helping yourself! You will simply gain the weight again, and that's not what fasting is about. Ease yourself into a meal and ensure that you're energizing yourself and are stated, but don't binge and eat unhealthily.

## Add Apple Cider Vinegar

Apple cider vinegar has been found to have many health benefits like clearing your gut, helping your digestion, and stabilizing your blood sugar. If you can, try and start or end your eating window with this drink so you can have an easier fasting period and gain these health benefits too. It will actually enhance your health goals and allow you to gain more benefits!

If you don't like the pungent taste of apple cider vinegar, there are even organic pills that you can take which give you the same benefits without the strong taste and odor!

## Consume Plenty Of Calories During The Eating Window

As we mentioned with the carnivore diet, there's no limit on how much you should be eating. Of course, you don't want to overeat, but you want to ensure you're eating enough to give you energy through your fasting window. You will be eating fewer calories in the day because you will be fasting, so ensure you aren't skimping on your meal and trying to limit your intake. Eat enough, so you don't feel weak or fatigued during your fasting period.

## Go To Bed

As we mentioned previously, sleep can make or break your mood, especially when you're fasting. That's why a nightly routine is important to help your body relax and have a restful sleep. Have a routine that clears your mind, ensure your sleeping environment is cool and dark, and avoid caffeine before bed. The more energized you feel the next day, the better you can tackle your fasting window.

## Listen To Your Body

You might feel tired or grouchy when you're fasting - that's perfectly normal just like it would be when you try a new diet. But if you become concerned about your health or feel seriously ill, it's important you stop fasting right away. Your health is the most important concern. If you feel unable to perform your daily tasks or feelings of sudden discomfort or pain, stop fasting right away and seek medical help.

## › RECAP

---

With our tips and tricks for success, you can learn what to do and not do when it comes to your fasting window. Keep yourself busy, stay hydrated, have some caffeine, and a good night's sleep. Don't binge on food after your fasting window is done, and always keep your health in mind if you need to stop fasting due to any pain.

## › ACTION ITEMS

---

Find which items you could implement in your fasting window to ensure it goes even more smoothly and safely for you.

# Chapter 10

# FAQ About Fasting, Autophagy, And The Carnivore Diet

Here are some frequently asked questions regarding fasting, autophagy, and the carnivore diet which are answered for you. With this information, you can make an informed decision about your health!

## Can't I Just Reduce Calories Instead?

No, not exactly.

Calorie reduction is changing what you're eating in a day or how much quantity of food you're eating. It doesn't say anything about when you eat in the day. With fasting, you're changing when you are eating throughout the day by giving yourself a fasting window to stick to - be that 12 hours, 16 hours or 20 hours. The research shows that fasting, or going without food for a period of time, is what can bring those potential health benefits. Calorie reduction can help you lose weight, but that doesn't mean it has other health benefits with it.

## What Are The Side Effects Of Fasting?

---

Just like when embarking on any possible diet change or lifestyle change, there may be possible side effects for you to deal with. These don't necessarily have to occur for you, but it's something to be aware of Side effects could include hunger pangs, headaches, constipation, weakness, dizziness or muscle cramps. These can occur as your body first adjusts to fasting and going without food for a longer amount of time. If you feel anything more severe than these symptoms, or any sort of pain or discomfort, be sure you stop fasting and seek medical help.

## How Do I Manage Hunger?

People often think of hunger like a wave that will overpower them or cripple them in the middle of the day. But that's not true! It might sneak up on you, but it doesn't have to sidetrack you completely. That's why it's important you're ready with hydration in the form of water, tea, or coffee, and that you keep yourself mentally and physically busy. Whether that's busy at work, reading, exercising, or relaxing, the more occupied you are, the smoother your fasting period may fast.

## There's No way I Can Fast For 24 Hours!

---

And that's okay!

Fasting is about finding what method works for you. If you don't feel up to fasting for that long, you don't have to. And you certainly shouldn't do it on your first try! Instead, first, see how close you are to completing a 12-hour fast and then try doing a 16-hour one. The more research you do and the more confident you are, the more surprised you will be at your strength and how your body adapts to changes.

## Do I Have To Stress My Body To Initiate Autophagy?

---

Autophagy can occur normally in the body, but it may take a longer amount of time for that to occur. During that time period, it means damaged or older cells are still in the immune system and functioning as a part of your cellular system. In order to initiate the process of autophagy to "clean up" your cells, you have to exert stress in the form of exercise or fasting. That's why the research shows that fasting can accelerate the rate of autophagy in the body and allow your immune system to perform faster.

## Isn't Too Much Protein Bad For You?

The carnivore diet is not an all protein diet. It is extremely low carbohydrate to the point of trying to avoid them, but more than 50% of it includes nutrients from fat. Compared to the ketogenic diet, it allows more flexibility where you can have a healthy balance of fat and protein. The keto diet allows for a minimum amount of carbohydrate but restricts protein to about 20% of your intake.

# Can I Use Spices To Flavor The Meat?

Sure!

No one expects you to eat raw meat!

Spices are great for seasoning your food and adding flavor, and they really have minuscule calorie counts. Experiment with fresh spices and the flavors of them so you can have a delicious meal. Turmeric, cayenne, black pepper, rosemary, and sage are all great in marinades and flavoring your food. It's also a great way to reduce your salt intake (although you do want to be sure you have enough salt in your diet to maintain an electrolyte balance). Salt, herbs, spices, and pepper are all allowed on the carnivore diet though you want to stay away from condiments that contain carbohydrates  If you find a zero-carb sauce, that would be allowed!

# Isn't The Carnivore Diet Expensive?

No, it doesn't have to be!

No matter what type of diet you eat, food quality should be important to you. With the carnivore diet, you are going to be shopping mainly for meat and animal-based products. But you also won't be spending money on other things like dessert, fruit, vegetables, or plant-based products you may have included on your shopping list before. So it really evens out! High-quality fats are not cheap, and you want to try and shop for organic or grass-fed meats when you can. You'll be saving money excluding other food groups from your shopping list so you can put that towards high-quality ingredients. Also, consider including organ meats and bones for bone broth. Those tend to be a little less expensive, and it's a great way to add variety to your diet.

Think of it as an investment. The more you put into your health now, the less you'll have to spend on doctor bills later.

## Eating Lots Of Meat Will Help Me Lose Weight?

The way that the carnivore diet helps you lose weight is by pushing your body into a process called ketosis. The reason this occurs is because of you cutting carbohydrates out of your diet. Without carbs, the body does not create glucose as a form of energy - it goes through ketosis to create molecules called "ketones" instead. Where do these ketones come from? They come from the fat our body already has stored away! That's right - we have the source of energy all along, but because we continue to eat carbohydrates in every meal, our body does not harness those ketones. By implementing the carnivore diet and also adding fasting to your routine, you are continually guiding your body towards ketosis to help you burn fat into the fuel you need.

Coupled with fasting, you'll become a fat burning machine.

# Are Eggs Allowed?

Absolutely!

Eggs are an animal-based protein.

Eggs have a great ratio of protein and fat to keep your body in balance. Not to mention that they are usually relatively inexpensive and very quick and easy to make! Whether it's scrambled eggs or a hard-boiled egg with your meal, they are perfect to include in the carnivore diet.

# Eating Meat And Fasting Will Give Me Mental Focus?

Yup, thanks to the power of ketosis, mental acuity skyrockets.

Ketosis is a type of fat that the body will be running on instead of glucose produced from the carbohydrates you would normally eat. Studies have shown that because these ketones are harvested from fat, they contain more energy and can give you a burst of physical and mental energy. Whether that's helping your performance at work or school, or giving you the energy to get through your workout at the gym, it's all about eating a diet low on carbohydrates to allow your body to produce ketones instead.

## Don't People Need Fruits And Vegetables?

The answer is not necessarily. In fact, red meat contains nearly every vitamin and mineral that your body needs - from vitamin D, protein, iron, vitamin B, and zinc! The only thing it doesn't have is vitamin C, but there's a lot of research supporting that you don't need vitamin C when you remove carbohydrates from your diet.

# Is It Dangerous To "Force" Autophagy?

No, because autophagy is a natural biological function of the body. It's there to help the body maintain equilibrium and to keep the body working smoothly. Think of it this way: the more you clean up your body's cellular system, the better it works for you. You're able to remove degraded cells, older cells not functioning as well, and possible mutated cells. This is better for your health! With the research proving an increased rate of autophagy could prevent neurodegenerative diseases and even cancer, why wouldn't you want to speed up the process?

## › RECAP

With your frequently asked questions answered, we are here to give you the facts about autophagy, the carnivore diet, and fasting! You will not become vitamin deficient on the carnivore diet, you don't have to count your macros on it, and you can still eat eggs and use spices and seasonings for your food!

# Conclusion

Thank you for making it to the end of *Fasting for the Carnivore Diet*. We hope that this book was helpful in answering your questions regarding fasting, autophagy, and the carnivore diet. There are many myths about fasting that have given it a bad reputation and labeled it as an "extreme" method of weight loss. But when we see the roots of fasting and the history behind it, it's easy to see how it was once a part of our ancestors' lives. Not only that, many world religions make it a point to include fasting in their calendar. For them, it's a way of atoning for sins or asking for forgiveness, but it shows that fasting is a perfectly reasonable act that you too can partake in!

With this book, we have hoped to show you some of the beneficial aspects of fasting and what the science behind fasting has proven. With this research, there has been a burst of new interest in fasting and the health benefits it provides. If you have a family history of diabetes and you are hoping to avoid medication and keep your blood sugar levels stable, fasting could be perfect for you. Do you want to lower your blood pressure and your cholesterol? Fasting can help with that too! What about having more energy and improving your mental focus and clarity? Believe it or not, eating less food can help you with having more energy! When we see what the research shows when implementing a routine of fasting in our lives, many people have found it a way to improve their health and maybe even extend their longevity.

The next step is to decide how fasting is something that you can include in your lifestyle. Whether you hope to do 12-hour or 16-hour fasts, it's important that you first do your research and figure out how you can make fasting work. Will you skip breakfast? Or do you prefer to skip dinner? How will you be keeping yourself busy to ensure you don't get tempted by food? What is your goal when you are fasting and giving up food? All these questions should be answered so you can have a successful fasting period. We hope we've provided you plenty of tips and tricks on how to get started and how to have a successful fast. From remembering your motivation to ensuring you aren't binging on calories, to keeping tea and coffee nearby, it's important you are armed with information to keep you confident and positive.

Finally, if you found this book useful in any way, a review is always appreciated!

# Thank You From Story Ninjas

Story Ninjas Publishing would like to thank you for reading this product. We hope you found value in our book and would love to hear your feedback. Please provide your constructive criticism in a review on Amazon. Also feel free to share this book with your friends through various social media platforms.

## Other Books by Story Ninjas

Story Ninjas Publishing hopes you enjoyed this book. You can find more of our products, by checking out our Amazon page.

## About Story Ninjas

Story Ninjas Publishing is an independent book publisher. Our stories range from science fiction to paranormal romance. Our goal is to create stories that are not only entertaining but endearing. We believe engaging narrative can lead to personal growth. Through unforgettable characters and a powerful plot, we portray themes that are relevant to today's issues. Our hope is that readers find lessons they can apply to their everyday lives so that the stories live on through the actions of each person they touch. Additionally, we provide creative non-fiction books that are meant to serve as tools to help people solve everyday problems. We hope you find our products entertaining and helpful.

You can find more Story Ninja's products here.

*Follow Story Ninjas!!!*
Website: www.Story-Ninjas.com
Email: Story-Ninjas@Story-Ninjas.com

Instagram: @StoryNinjas
Facebook: StoryNinjasHQ
LinkedIn: Story-Ninjas
Blogger: Story-NinjasHQ
Twitter: @StoryNinjas
Youtube: @StoryNinjas
Amazon: Story Ninjas
Podcast: Polymathics

Made in the USA
San Bernardino, CA
15 June 2019